DREAMS

JOHNS HOPKINS
UNIVERSITY PRESS

AARHUS UNIVERSITY PRESS

dream

MELANIE
GILLESPIE ROSEN

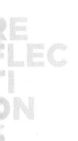

DREAMS

© Melanie Gillespie Rosen
and Johns Hopkins University Press 2023
Layout and cover: Camilla Jørgensen, Trefold
Cover photograph: Poul Ib Henriksen
Publishing editor: Karina Bell Ottosen
Translated from the Danish by Heidi Flegal
Printed by Narayana Press, Denmark
Printed in Denmark 2023

ISBN 978-1-4214-4712-4 (pbk)
ISBN 978-1-4214-4713-1 (ebook)

Library of Congress Control Number: 2022949357

*Special discounts are available for bulk purchases of this
book. For more information, please contact Special Sales at
specialsales@jh.edu.*

Published in the United States by:

Johns Hopkins University Press
2715 North Charles Street
Baltimore, MD 21218
www.press.jhu.edu

Published with the generous support of the
Aarhus University Research Foundation

Purchase in Denmark: ISBN 978-87-7219-285-7

Aarhus University Press
Helsingforsgade 25
8200 Aarhus N
Denmark
www.aarhusuniversitypress.dk

PEER
REVIEWED

MIX
Paper
FSC FSC® C010651

CONTENTS

DISTURBING NOCTURNAL ACTIVITY

AN UNSETTLING EXPERIENCE

You're sitting at your desk minding your own business when, out of nowhere, your mother appears. She's wearing that orange clown suit she only wears for special occasions. She's obviously angry – steam is coming out of her ears. What should you do? She is rapidly turning into a lion and you know that when the transformation is complete, you're toast. Perhaps, if you try very hard, you can fly away and save yourself. On good days you can fly quite well, after all. But not today. Right now you're so distracted by your impending doom that you can't even levitate. The lion pounces. You throw your hands up and try to protect your face ...

... and find yourself sitting up in bed. Your hands *are* in front of you. You're sweating, breathing heavily, and your heart racing ... It takes you a few seconds to reorient yourself and realise where you are. Whew! It was just a dream, and a weird one at that. What a vivid and amazing experience. It felt so real, but it was so very strange. And yet, within seconds, the whole experience starts to drain away from your mind until you can barely remember a thing. You're sure you had a dream, but what was it about? You can no longer say.

What happened? One minute you think you are awake and at work. It feels so real until, suddenly, things get seriously weird. Even then, you don't realise anything is out of the ordinary. Bizarre, even impossible events transpire and you think they are all totally normal. You even experience some false memories, *thinking* that you remember an event although it never actually happened. To your delusional mind, these explain away the weirdness: your mother's clown suit, and your own attempt to fly away.

Perhaps even more amazing is the fact that you felt like you were moving around and upright when, in reality, your body was completely paralysed and lying down. Your eyes were shut, yet you could see. For something like this to happen seems so incredible, a full-on hallucination, and yet moments after waking you usually forget nearly everything. At other times, you manage to remember the dream and make a *dream report* – you tell your partner about it, write it down in a dream diary or bore your friends with it. Perhaps you think dreams are all meaningless nonsense. Or perhaps you think they tell you something important about yourself, even the really weird ones. Especially the weird ones. You might just find dreaming fun to do. I am not here to tell you whether you are right or wrong about your own dreams. However, the fact that we dream at all, I think you will agree, is itself quite incredible.

A MYSTERY IN THE NIGHT

Dreams have puzzled philosophers for millennia. Earlier than 300 BCE, the ancient Greek philosopher Aristotle theorised that dreams were caused by the sense organs continuing to move after falling asleep. René Descartes, a French philosopher of the 1600s, thought that dreams were so profound and realistic they gave us reason to be sceptical about whether the external world existed. He reasoned that sometimes we need to wake up from a dream to realise it was a dream. If I need to wake up before knowing whether it was a dream, I might be dreaming right now. This means I may have been deceived into thinking the external world really exists when it's all just a dream, so I don't *know* it exists for sure. But at least *I* must exist to be deceived in the first place. As long as I am thinking, at least I know that I exist. This is the origin of one of the most famous philosophical sayings of all time: *Cogito ergo sum* – "I think, therefore, I am."

It was not until the early 1950s that the first major scientific breakthrough about dreams was made, when the American neurologists Eugene Aserinsky and Nathaniel Kleitman discovered 'rapid eye movement' sleep. They initially thought they had discovered a sleep stage in which all dreams occur. The American philosopher Norman Malcolm was not convinced, however. He found dreams so baffling that in the late 1950s, he responded to these new scientific findings with the most sceptical argument since Descartes. He argued that we do not, in fact, dream at all. Rather, we simply make up stories when we wake up.

Who is right? Thousands of years after Aristotle, we are still baffled. According to some current researchers, Aristotle was not too far off after all, although exactly how the body relates to our dreams is still up for debate. Malcolm, on the other hand, was totally wrong: humans most definitely dream. And what about Descartes? Well, we cannot actually know whether the external world exists. You may have seen *The Matrix*, a film from 1999 that popularised the idea that we may all be living in a computer program controlled by robots. Although this idea seems very unlikely, how can we know for sure?

According to the modern American philosopher Eric Schwitzgebel, there are a few possible but extremely unlikely situations in which the external world does not exist. Dreaming is one, but we are unlikely to be dreaming now, because when we think about whether or not we are dreaming, we can usually tell. If I were dreaming right now, I could look around to try to find something unusual. Dreams are usually different from the waking world, so to notice the difference, we need to pay attention. I could try to levitate. If I succeed, it's a dream for sure. In this scenario, I would be *lucid dreaming*, which is when we realise that we are dreaming during a dream. But right now everything looks very normal and I have no special powers of levitation, so I'm fairly sure I'm awake.

The *Matrix* scenario is much less likely than the possibility that we are dreaming. We have no reason to think that the world we see is actually a computer program, although that does not mean it is impossible. Perhaps a mad scientist or, as Descartes pondered, an evil demon is fooling us using technology we do not know about, or magic. Once again, this is highly unlikely but not entirely impossible. This results in a very low likelihood that the external world does not exist. We will just have to be satisfied with being 99.9% sure about the external world, or 0.1% sceptical of it.

Modern philosophers and scientists have been working on several difficult questions about dreaming that remain unresolved. Why do we have dreams? What, if any, is their evolutionary purpose? Do my dreams reveal anything about me as a person? More fundamentally, what *are* dreams? And what does it feel like to dream?

THE STUFF DREAMS ARE MADE OF

DO YOU REALLY KNOW WHAT YOU THINK YOU KNOW?

We all think we know what it means to dream. Dreams are experiences we have after we fall asleep and before we wake up again. They seem real when we are having them, and in most dreams we believe we are awake, so perhaps they are best described as realistic hallucinations. They are mostly visual. Have you ever tried to pinch yourself while you were dreaming? You probably didn't feel anything, so you may think that dreams are *only* visual. But someone else might experience dreams differently. Some of us even feel pain while dreaming, so dreams cannot be exclusively visual. They can certainly include sounds, and you might hear music, talking, wind in the trees … the possibilities are endless. In my own dreams, on occasion I have tasted cakes and chocolates, and smelled fragrances and foul odours.

TECHNICOLOURED OR MONOCHROME?

What about colour? Some people report dreaming in black and white, while others experience bright technicoloured scenes or anything in between. Some theorists have claimed that dreams are bizarre and weird, whereas others deny that this is true, claiming instead that most dreams are, in fact, quite mundane. We tend to remember the weird ones and forget the boring ones. If we run a controlled experiment in a lab where a sleeping person is woken up at different times during the night, they are actually likely to report excruciatingly dull dreams. Instead of lion attacks, we dream about tedious tasks at work. What a waste of dream time.

Scientists have also discovered that we dream much more than we think we do. This might sound ironic, but I hardly ever remember a dream when I wake up, only once every few months. I spend all day researching dreams, but I seem to have hardly any of my own. How sad. A lot of people share my situation, but this doesn't mean we don't dream very much. We just don't remember them. When scientists wake people up and have them report their dreams right away, memory improves considerably. If people are woken up during the rapid eye movement or 'REM' stage of sleep – when the eyes move around erratically beneath the eyelids – 80–90% of the time they will remember a dream. Since most adults have five or six REM sessions per night, we could be having at least that many dreams. It is difficult to determine how long we spend dreaming each night, but a fair estimate is that dreams take up a quarter of our sleep time.

Dreams can also occur in other sleep stages. Sleep is usually divided into four stages, three of which are non-rapid eye movement or 'NREM', which, as one would expect from the name, do not have the same eye movements. During stages 1 and 2, the light stages of sleep, the eyes move, but they are slower than during REM sleep. In these stages, our bodies start to relax although they occasionally twitch. Electrical brain activation slows down, so that by the time we reach stage 3, or 'deep sleep', the brain waves are very slow 'delta' waves. It is quite difficult to wake a person from this stage of sleep. In contrast, REM sleep has wake-like brain activity, known as 'gamma' waves. While it does makes sense that dreams occur when the brain is at its most active, it turns out that dreams can actually occur during REM *and* NREM sleep, although they are less common in NREM stages.

People who do not dream at all are very rare, and the condition is usually caused by a brain injury. It seems that people who do not dream but still have REM sleep do not suffer any serious ill effects, as opposed to people who do not sleep. Disorders such as 'fatal familial insomnia', which, starting in mature adulthood, prevents sufferers from sleeping at all, invariably lead to insanity, coma and ultimately death some months after the symptoms start. Unlike with sleeping, even if I had never dreamt, I would probably be fine. However, most people who believe they do not dream simply fail to remember them, which is easily proven by waking them up during REM.

This means that I dream much more than I remember, and the kinds of dreams I do remember are probably not a good indication of what all dreams, or even most dreams, are like. This brings us no closer to saying exactly what dreams are. However, because they are so varied it is easier to start by looking at what dreams are *not*.

MAKING UP STORIES

Firstly, dreams are not just stories we make up when we wake up, as Malcolm thought, although we may sometimes do this. Malcolm observed that we cannot report dreams while we are having them, and our sleeping bodies do not move around or act out our dreams. Someone watching us sleep cannot see what we are experiencing. Normally the only way we can know about what someone is experiencing is by their reports and behaviour, but since dreams can only be reported after the fact, they cannot be verified the same way as our waking experiences can. This scepticism about our own experiences is somewhat similar to Descartes' scepticism about the external world. But where Descartes used dreams to be sceptical about waking experience, Malcolm instead argued that we should be entirely sceptical about dreams: we can only verify that a report is made, so that is all dreams are.

For anyone who has ever remembered a dream, which is nearly everyone, it seems preposterous to claim that dreams are just stories we make up, and that no sleep experiences really happen. I know for a fact that I'm not just making these stories up. Or do I? As odd as this view may sound, the celebrated American philosopher of mind Daniel Dennett proposed a theory that dreams are *false memories* that are stored in the mind and replayed upon waking. This means that we *believe* we experienced something while asleep, but never really did. How can anyone tell the difference between a real memory and a false memory? If we want to check whether a memory is true, we can usually ask someone who remembers the same event, check the photos or think about how likely it was that the event actually occured. But with dreams, none of this applies. No one else was there, there are no photos or videos, and dreams can be entirely unrealistic, so there is no way to check them for plausibility. It is also likely that our dream memories change quite a lot on retelling. The sceptical theories of Malcolm and Dennett brought about a new interest in dreaming at the time and generated quite a heated debate. How might we disprove this scepticism?

Well, just as we cannot be 100% sure that the external world really exists, we cannot be 100% sure that our memories are true. Even so, we can be *quite* sure that, at least some of the time, we really do have experiences while we're asleep. One very good reason to think this is that we can learn to become 'lucid' or aware of the fact that we are dreaming. When this occurs, we can actually signal to experimenters with eye flicks. These can be measured by a technique called electrooculography, or EOG, which uses electrodes to measure the twitches of the eye muscles. Flicking the eyes left, right, left, right in a dream usually causes the dreamer's real eyes to do the same thing, and EOG picks up the signals. This experiment has been repeated many times, disproving Malcolm's view that people can never 'report' a dream while it is happening –

provided, of course, that we acknowledge that such signals are indeed a report that says 'I am dreaming'.

WHAT A RELIEF TO BE PARALYSED AT NIGHT

Another strong reason to reject Malcolm's view is a condition known as 'REM sleep behaviour disorder', in which people act out their dreams. This is not the same as sleepwalking, where a sleeping person walks around and is usually quite safe. Sleepwalking normally occurs half-way between waking and sleeping. Sleepwalkers can avoid bumping into tables and chairs, and can even walk down stairs. On the other hand, it is very dangerous when a person actually acts out their dreams. Dreaming about diving into a pool would cause serious injury if acted out.

REM sleep behaviour disorder can injure to or even kill the dreamer or people in their vicinity, especially their partner. Why does this happen? Usually, we become paralysed during REM sleep. Several neurological conditions, including Parkinson's disease, can damage the part of the brain stem that causes this paralysed state. This is a dangerous condition to have, but it disproves Malcolm's view that it is impossible for a sleeping person to display behaviour – some people do indeed move about and act out what they are experiencing in their dream.

We can conclude from this that experiences do happen during sleep. The next question is, what kind of experiences? Just because we know that dreams *do* occur, that does not mean we can trust all dream reports. Dreams are notoriously hard to remember. We might get the details wrong, and since no one other than the dreamer can see what is going on, potential mistakes cannot be corrected.

Even if we can trust certain reports, researchers disagree on how to measure their content. One example is the debate about whether dreams are bizarre or mundane. To determine just how weird dreams are, researchers have designed 'bizarreness scales' to classify each item in a dream report. They then rate how many bizarre items occur in comparison to the total length of the report. One of the problems with this method is that different research groups use different scales, which give different answers.

Some rating scales include two categories, for instance *how* bizarre something is – whether it is 'unusual', 'fantastical' or 'impossible' – and *what* content is involved – typically 'persons', 'objects' or 'places'. An example of a 'fantastical object' would be a magic wand, while my friend suddenly having purple hair would be an 'unusual person'. However, you could operate with more or fewer categories, or specify different types of content. Should thoughts be included? How many distinctive degrees of bizarreness should a scale have? This has not been standardised.

Different scales mean that research groups may find different levels of bizarreness. And there is another aspect of this research that I find problematic: to avoid bias, which might result from analysts knowing too much about the study subjects, bizarreness assessors know nothing about the dreamer.

BIZARRENESS IS IN THE EYE OF THE BEHOLDER

When experiments are done on human subjects, researchers who analyse the results are usually 'blinded' and receive no details about those subjects. This is to avoid bias or undue influence on the researchers, who otherwise may tend towards a particular result from knowing too much about the subjects who report their dreams. One common bias is that when we expect a certain result, we are more likely to find that result, whether it is true or not.

Let us apply this to dreams using a fictitious example: if I expect men's dreams to be more bizarre than women's dreams, and if I know which reports come from men, I might be more likely to notice bizarre elements in these reports. As I mentioned, to avoid bias, the people analysing the dreams do not know anything about the dreamers. However, this method is problematic in bizarreness research because what counts as bizarre is subjective and very individual. What is bizarre to me may not be to you at all, and vice versa. Dreaming about working in an office is quite normal for me, but it would be bizarre had I never worked in an office. Blinded assessors would not know about these nuances, so they might consider some elements as bizarre that are common to the dreamer in question, or regard others as normal that ought to be assessed as bizarre. This means that bizarreness measures can be inaccurate.

Bizarreness in dreams is highly diverse. They can be entirely fantastical and impossible, involving magic, dragons, and levitating, or totally mundane and normal, about working or doing everyday tasks. I therefore maintain that we cannnot simply define all dreams as 'bizarre' or 'mundane', since they can be anywhere on what we might call a 'weirdness spectrum'.

A slightly different issue is whether dreams are very realistic. This differs from bizarreness, given that a boring dream may still not be realistic, as when a room looks blurry or 'dreamy' and feels unreal. It may not feel like you are really there, more like you are watching a boring movie than walking around your office. *Realistic* would denote a vivid, convincing experience that involves multiple senses and makes the dreamer feel either awake or at least in a realistic virtual reality. A person can also have a bizarre but realistic dream. This is a complicated issue, as it ties into whether we are stupid when we are dreaming, or whether we could be just as smart as we are when awake.

People often report thinking a dream was real until they wake up and find themselves in bed. Does this mean dreams *are* realistic? Not necessarily. If we fail to pay attention to our surroundings, then we might not notice when they are unrealistic. Researchers have found evidence that people can be quite idiotic when dreaming. We do not notice weirdness, we make bad decisions and we act strangely. But as with bizarreness, I don't think that these cognitive failings occur in all dreams. We can be quite intelligent, as we can see from lucid dreams, where we realise we are dreaming and can carry out quite complex tasks and even participate in eye-signalling experiments.

Could we be even smarter in a dream than when we are awake?

QUIET PLEASE: GENIUS ASLEEP

It has not been proven that people can have a stroke of genius in a dream, but it is possible, as many celebrated cases of dream inspiration indicate. Artists ranging from musicians to painters have been inspired by their dreams. Perhaps the most well-known example is the Spanish painter, Salvador Dalí, who famously rendered scenes from his dreams. Even so, that does not mean he was a genius in his dreams. Dalí was an expert painter who, while awake, depicted amazing images from dreams, all of which are quite bizarre – like most of the dreams the rest of us remember.

What about other types of genius? The German pharmacologist Otto Loewi dreamt about an experiment that would show whether nerve impulses were electrical or chemical. He woke up and tried out the experiment, and it worked, proving that the impulses were, in fact, chemical. Thirteen years later, in 1936, Loewi won a Nobel Prize for his discovery. This seems amazing and somewhat far-fetched. How do we know whether this account is mere myth? In these legendary examples it is very hard to discern the truth. However, perhaps you've had an experience like this yourself, or know someone who has. I don't mean that you found you were better at solving a problem after a good night's sleep, which may happen simply because your brain is well rested. What I mean is that you had a dream which actually solved a specific problem.

I chatted with the American philosopher Jonathan Ichikawa after a conference once, and he told me about a 'smart dream' he once had. As a university undergraduate he was given a logic problem to solve. During the day he came up with a poor solution, but that night, in a dream, he came up with a far better one. When he woke up, he double-checked his answer and it worked. Because I heard the dream report directly from the person who had the dream, I trust Ichikawa's report than the celebrated cases where there is no first-hand testimony. As surprising as this is, apparently sometimes we can indeed be very smart in our dreams, bearing in mind that dreams are extremely varied and that we are far more likely to be stupid.

In dreams we can, at times, be cognitively impaired, whereas sometimes we can be even smarter than when we are awake. Dreams can be unrealistic or tremendously realistic. Exactly what percentage of dreams have these features is very difficult to know, due to several complexities. One is that different sleep stages give rise to different kinds of dreams. Early dream researchers, including the Americans neurologists Eugene Aserinsky and Nathaniel Kleitman – who discovered REM sleep – first thought that dreams only occurred during REM. We now know they were wrong about this, although dreams are far more common during this stage. We also know that dreams differ greatly over the course of a night.

As we are first drifting off, our minds start to wander

and our thoughts can be weird or repetitive. Perhaps these experiences should not be counted as dreams, since they are just relaxed imagining or 'mind-wandering', but these thoughts can become quite vivid and detailed. Then, as we start to sink into sleep stage 1, we can have very vivid sensations, such as the feeling of falling, known as 'hypnagogic hallucinations'. I often sit up in bed with my hands thrown in front of me, thinking I'm falling off my bicycle. What is probably happening is a mix of detailed, vivid mind-wandering about bike riding, and then a hypnagogic hallucination of falling which I put together in my mind. Whether this should be called 'dreaming' or not seems somewhat arbitrary. However, if we say that these episodes are not really dreams, perhaps some of the other experiences we have in sleep should not be considered to be dreams either? Nevertheless, it is hard to deny that at least some of the experiences that occur in NREM sleep are real dreams, and they can be quite similar in content to REM-sleep dreams.

ALL NIGHT LONG

Compared to REM dreams, NREM dreams, especially in sleep stages 1 and 2, are rarer and usually less vivid, involve less intense sensations and are more likely to be thought-like or imagination-like than perceptual. Dreams in stages 1 and 2 might be more like being in a dark room with your eyes closed and just letting your mind wander.

Experiments led by the American psychologist David Foulkes in the 1970s on people having exactly this kind of experience surprisingly showed that mind-wandering can be quite vivid and immersive. Some people even forget they are mind-wandering, so perhaps the difference between imagination and hallucination is not so clear after all. Yet one thing that is quite clear is that people who are woken up from REM sleep report their state as much more 'immersive', meaning they feel they are *in* the dream which is realistic, convincing and lifelike. These dreams can be described as similar to virtual reality.

The dreams we have during REM sleep are by far the most memorable. Perhaps this is because they are the most vivid and interesting, or perhaps our memory is better during this stage. So, if you think all dreams are bizarre, that may just be because you only remember the bizarre ones. Despite this, no matter how bizarre a dream is, we are still quite unlikely to recall it. Do you consider your dream memory to be good? Much better than mine? Well, even if you remember two dreams every night, which is rare indeed, you're still forgetting more than half. On the other hand, if you're like me, you're forgetting five or more dreams per night. This really is quite a shame. So many of my dream experiences, some of them quite fantastical and amazing, are forgotten instantly. If only I could remember more.

THE SCIENTIFIC STUDY OF DREAMS

WHY BOTHER?

Dreams are notoriously difficult to study. At a recent conference I met an established dream researcher who recommended that, for this very reason, young cognitive scientists and neuroscientists should wait until they get an established, permanent job before moving into dream research. Oops: I got into the field too early! Luckily, I'm a philosopher, and I don't have to deal with running troublesome experiments. But what's so hard about dream science anyway?

Recent research has improved our understanding of dreams thanks to hours of tireless study, new techniques, innovation and technology. However, despite all of this modern technology, studying dreams remains very difficult. One could argue that all science is hard, which is certainly true. But there is an added layer of difficulty in studying dreams compared to studying waking experiences. If you want to do scientific research on, for example, how people see an image when they are awake, you can control what a subject is looking at, track their eyes, look at their brain activation using a variety of scanners and ask them what they are experiencing at any stage of the experiment.

I am not saying this is easy. It takes years of training, experience, expensive equipment, and lots of researchers and funding, and still mistakes can be made or the findings could be inconsequential. Participants may not respond the way they are expected to at all. But now, think about what would be required to do an experiment on what a sleeping person sees. Sure, we can get a subject to fall asleep in a lab and hook them up to fancy, expensive equipment, track eye movements, and look at bodily twitches and brain activation, just as we do with waking participants. The equipment can be noisy and uncomfortable, making it hard to sleep, but it can certainly be done. We can then wake the sleeper to ask whether they were dreaming and, if so, what their dream was about. The researchers record the dreamers' reports and can then see what their brains and bodies were doing during the dream. However, this is even more difficult than a waking experiment.

A subject wakes up and reports a dream. How do experimenters know precisely when during the night the dream occurred? We can have multiple dreams a night, after all. It most likely occurred right before the dreamer awoke, but it is hard to know for sure. Timing is crucial for neuroimaging studies, which rely on comparing dream reports with records of brain activation. It is also difficult to know what brain activation is occurring during a specific part of a dream. The problem here is that we must wake dreamers up, then ask them about their dream; we cannot simply ask them while it is happening, which would be much better. Researchers could try asking a sleeping person what they are experiencing, but the only response they would get is snoring. The more time passes, the more we forget, both when we are awake and when we are dreaming, yet the latter is much more problematic because dreamers are particularly forgetful.

All of us – even those with the best memories – forget most of our dreams. One explanation for this is that major electrical activation and chemical changes occur in the brain during sleep which leads to poor memory. A neurotransmitter called norepinephrine, which is key to memory retention, is severely reduced during dreaming compared to when we are awake. Parts of the brain implicated in the generation of memories, such as the prefrontal cortex, generally show reduced activation. This is why, no matter how outlandish a dream is, when you wake up it tends to drain away from your mind within seconds. However, if we manage to hold on to a dream memory for a few minutes while the brain shifts back into the wake state, which has higher prefrontal activation and increased norepinephrine, the memory can be retained. This can require considerable mental effort and a retelling of the dream story.

The impossiblilty of reporting dreams while they are happening and our very poor memories of the dreams we have make dream science more difficult. Another issue is that researchers have virtually no control over what their dreaming subjects experience – bearing in mind that scientists love to have every experimental variable under control.

If we want to study how people see a certain image while awake and what their brain is doing at the time, we can just get a subject to look at the image while they are in a scanner. In dream research this is not an option.

People's dreams really are quite random and unpredictable, but imagine that we wanted to see what brain activation goes on when someone is flying in a dream. It is extremely difficult to plan to make such a dream occur, but there are methods we can use. One is to get an 'expert' lucid dreamer, a person who has learned how to lucid dream and can do it regularly, to try to control their dream in the way the experimenter asks. This technique has been used by quite a few researchers, but one problem is that there are some differences between average lucid and non-lucid dreams. This means we cannot always use lucid dreams as a stand-in for regular dreaming. Also, it is not easy to collect a large sample of reports about lucid dreaming. Many expert lucid dreamers need to attempt the experiment over many nights, sometimes with little success. What is more, because we rely so heavily on reports to investigate dreams scientifically, it is also difficult to know whether animals and humans who cannot talk, such as babies and fetuses, have dreams.

A GOOD MIND TO DREAM?

I know that I have dreams because I remember them when I wake up. I know about your dreams if you choose to tell me about them. Researchers know that most human adults dream because of experiments showing that nearly every adult reports dreams when woken from REM sleep, and sometimes also from other stages. But do babies dream too? Fetuses? Animals? Trees? Well, trees probably don't. But what about animals in general, or particular species? What might their dreams be like, if they have any? We really do not know.

Many of us have been amused to see our dog or cat twitching in their sleep. It looks like they are dreaming of chasing a stick or playing with a toy. But do we really know? They are unable to tell us. And as for humans, when do we even start dreaming? Recent research suggests that fetuses undergo REM-like sleep stages from 7 months' gestation and at this stage, brain activity appears to be about as complex as that of a conscious brain. If this is true, then surely some animals are able to dream too? Yet the mere fact that fetuses and animals have REM sleep does not necessarily mean they also dream.

The American psychologist David Foulkes does not think animals, fetuses or even young children dream. He believes that children only start to dream when they are a few years old. The kind of immersive dreams that adults have start around age 7, according to Foulkes. This is because the cognitive mechanisms underlying our ability to dream, one of which is the ability to imagine, are not sufficiently developed until then. If this is true, then animals would also have to possess the ability to imagine for them to be able to dream. It is not clear whether animals *do* imagine in the way required. If not, this would suggest they do not dream either. Then again, if they do not, then why do they twitch in their sleep? The explanation might, instead, be an unconscious reactivation of motor processes or muscle memory.

We honestly do not know, which leaves many unanswered questions: Is the ability to imagine really necessary for the ability to dream? What if animals and fetuses are simply reactivating some of their waking, conscious experiences like the gentle light, warmth and pulsing sound of the womb's environment for the unborn baby and the joy of knocking over your favourite glass vase for the cat? Do animals and fetuses even have the kind of conscious experiences that could be reproduced as conscious dreams? We do not yet know the neural correlates of consciousness, meaning that we cannot just look at brain activation and determine whether a given animal is conscious, so an answer to this last question is a long way off. For now, we are obliged to focus dream research on those who can verbally report their dreams to us.

DREAM BODY

Aristotle lived in Athens a few thousand years before the modern scientific method was conceived, so we cannot expect him to have known much about the human body. Indeed, he thought the brain was a cooling system for the blood, and that our consciousness and intelligence were housed in the heart. He certainly knew nothing about REM sleep. He was right about a few things though. Apparently, a lot of what we dream about does relate to the real body, as Aristotle hypothesised. Very astute – and not bad for a proto-scientist and lowly philosopher. We have now confirmed the correlation thanks to experiments in which the human body is stimulated during REM sleep. They show that different sensations from external sources can actually be experienced by the dreamer. This is something you can safely try to replicate at home, provided you can get a willing subject to volunteer.

First, choose the stimulus you will use on your sleeping subject: spray water onto their face, shine a light in their eyes, apply pressure to their arm or play gentle music or sounds. Wait a minute, then wake them up so they can give you a dream report. Researchers would set this up in a dream lab and make sure the subject was in REM sleep to obtain the best results, but you can try applying the stimulus at any sleep stage. Quite often, dreamers report experiencing the stimulus within the dream, although certain stimuli are more likely to be felt than others. Light and sound are much less likely to enter the dream than pressure stimulus, for example. Having said that, it is very unlikely that every experience in a dream is caused this way. The things that appear to us in dreams can be extremely complex, which is unlikely to be caused by real visual stimuli. Light has a very low likelihood of being seen or incorporated into a dream, and even when it does register, it has to filter through our closed eyelids. A picture or a detailed image from a TV screen held in front of the dreamer's face would not be seen, so it seems that most of what we see in dreams is likely to be generated by the mind alone, not by real stimuli. And Aristotle? Well, at least he got some of it right.

The question is enormously interesting to philosophers, who have long debated whether a mind can experience anything while the brain is in a 'vat'. This refers to a science fiction thought experiment in which a brain is removed from a skull and put into a large container of nutrient liquid that keeps it alive – which is not quite like the *Matrix* scenario, in which the characters had their brains stimulated using complex futuristic technology. Rather, the thought experiment simply involves a live brain that has no stimulation from the outside at all. Dreaming could be a situation similar to the hypothetical brain in a vat.

OPEN AND CLOSED MINDS

Although, fortunately, our brains are not deposited in a jar of liquid when we sleep, the old way of thinking about dreams was that they are largely 'shut off' from the environment. The influential American psychiatrist J. Allan Hobson called this an 'input blockade'. Scientists and philosophers now agree that the mind is not completely shut off from the environment while dreaming, nor is it completely open to stimulus. We do not yet know exactly *how* open it is, and whether this changes across different sleep stages. It is likely that the mind is sometimes quite open, and at other times completely shut off. Otherwise, why would some stimuli make it into our dreams and some not?

We do not know the conditions under which openness occurs, or what factors cause it to vary, so it is a contentious topic. Some researchers, like Hobson, say that the dreaming mind is almost completely under an input blockade and shut off, with only the occasional stimulus getting in. Those on the other side of the spectrum, including Jennifer Windt, a German philosopher of mind and dreams, argue that dreams should generally be regarded as illusions of real stimuli – which would require that we quite regularly experience real stimuli while we sleep.

My own view is that the mind shifts between being more or less open in different stages of sleep, not only in the different main sleep stages, but also within sub-stages of REM sleep. Research suggests that there are at at least two such sub-stages, known as the 'tonic stage' and 'phasic stage'. While the phasic stage is likely to be much more open, the tonic stage is probably much more closed. This may sound complicated, but the full story is far more complex still, involving subtle shifts in brain activity that lead to different degrees of 'openness', which, for several reasons, is very difficult to test.

To be able to determine how open we are to dream stimulus, we would need very accurate tests to show when stimulus had been felt in a dream, and such tests do not exist. Since people have such a bad memory for dreams, just because someone cannot remember feeling a stimulus does not mean they didn't feel it at the time. Perhaps they just forgot about that particular sensation. This means stimulus might be under-reported. Another issue is that experimenters must interpret dream reports to work out whether a given stimulus had been felt. However, I may well dream that I see a red stop sign at the very moment an experimenter flashes a red light in my eyes, but the timing may be pure coincidence. Or perhaps I had a dream earlier in the night about something red, which I remember when I wake up, potentially leading to stimulus being over-reported. As I said, dream research really is quite hard.

Despite the difficulties, you can see why scientists are still drawn to dreams, which are fascinating and mystifying. As I already mentioned, I'm a philosopher, so I don't conduct experiments myself. Rather, I analyse other people's scientific research and use their findings to come up with theories about dreams. This means I am spared a good deal of worry about funding, participants and lab space. I never cease to be impressed by the creativity of dream scientists. Many recent experiments, especially those looking into lucid dreams, are incredibly sophisticated and awesomely innovative. Devising novel techniques, researchers are just starting to find ways to speak to dreamers when they are asleep, and even to look at brains and read dream content directly. These experiments usually apply established technology in new ways. And there are still many gaps in our knowledge that call for further innovation, so if you're creative and interested in science, dream research may be just the field for you.

ULTIMATE POWER AND FREEDOM

Many people, academics and non-academics alike, are intrigued by lucid dreams. Who would not want to realise they are dreaming during a dream? If you become lucid while dreaming, you can usually also gain control of the dream, which means you can do pretty much anything you like. You could never have that kind of control in your normal life. This control is also what draws researchers to the study of lucid dreams, and their work has led to some truly fascinating discoveries.

Teaching lucid-dreaming subjects to perform specific eye flicks during a dream, as I described earlier, was one of the first methods scientists invented to enable actual communication with dreamers. Before this technique was invented, some researchers even went so far as to deny that lucid dreams ever occurred. They thought that realising you were dreaming *during* a dream was just not possible. Today we know it is. Some expert lucid dreamers can become lucid regularly, multiple times per night, which is highly useful for research purposes. They usually carry out a simple eye-movement pattern – flick 'left, right, left, right', for instance – which anyone could do. It's harder, however, to remember to do this when they become lucid. On top of this, electroencephalography, or EEG, must be used to measure the subject's electrical brain activity to determine which stage of sleep they are in to make sure they are not half asleep or still awake.

As I described earlier, EOG measures the subject's eye movements but not the specifics, such as direction, so it can pick up a pattern of four flicks but is unable to register 'up, down, left, right'. But although the EOG method cannot determine direction, the eye movements can be matched up with the arm movements, as when a specific arm twitches and the eye flicks at the same time. These movements can then be matched up with dream reports.

One truly groundbreaking experiment was carried out in the 1980s on an expert dreamer who was trained to draw large letters on the ground while dreaming and track these movements with his eyes. Using electrodes to measure muscle twitches, the researchers found that the arm that was writing the letters in the dream would twitch in response to the dream movements. The dreamer could therefore communicate with the researchers while the dream was happening. These measurements allowed researchers to observe behaviour that indicated what was happening in the dream, which is a way of verifying the content of the dream.

SAVOURING A DREAM SANDWICH

Based on these and other innovations, scientists have more recently come up with new methods to find answers to some of the questions we have about dreams. Do people experience time differently in their dreams? To test this, researchers got expert lucid dreamers to carry out activities, such as doing a squat or counting, and using eye flicks to indicate the start and end of the activity. It turns out that people count at about the same speed in dreams and when awake, whereas, on average, doing physical activities takes a bit longer in a dream.

Other pioneering research, conducted by the French neurologist Isabelle Arnulf and colleagues, video-documents people with REM sleep behaviour disorder, or RBD, which causes them to act out their dreams. Sometimes one can clearly discern the dream from the dreamer's actions, which can be compared to waking actions. Unsurprisingly, but nonetheless fascinatingly, eating a dream sandwich does not take as long as eating a real sandwich. I suppose that's because there's a lot more chewing to do when the sandwich is real. I sometimes have dreams about eating and of course I never feel full either, no matter how much I stuff my face.

The ability of lucid dreamers to indicate that they are dreaming can be considered as a type of one-way communication from the dreamer to the researcher. Imagine that, as a scientist, you designed an excellent set-up that also enabled one-way communication from the experimenter to the dreamer using stimuli such as arm squeezes, flashing lights or recorded messages.

Recently, several research groups in different countries have tried to achieve two-way communication between dreamer and experimenter. The German cognitive scientist Kristoffer Appel used some relatively simple technology, including EEG, which measures general changes in electrical activity in the brain, and EOG, which measures eye movements using electrodes that sense muscle twitches. He then combined this established technology with more cutting-edge machine learning and brain–computer interfacing. Appel first played recorded questions to the sleeping person on repeat, doing so until they could hear the question and respond with eye flicks. Machine learning was then used so a computer program could pick up the signals from the EEG and EOG machines.

With some technological improvements, this sort of research could be done at subjects' homes rather than in the lab. The simplest communication would ask 'yes/no' questions and dreamers then respond with eye flicks to indicate their answers, but a more complicated system of flicks could be designed for more complex communication. If we pursue this line of research, eventually dreamers could be able to report their dreams as they happen.

FOR YOUR EYES ONLY

People often tell each other about their dreams, but some are too embarrassing to share. Wouldn't it be terrible if someone could watch your dream as it happened? The scariest dream experiment I can think of involves interpreting our dreams using brain-scan imaging. This may be your worst nightmare too, but not to worry: For now, your dreams are safe from prying eyes … unless, of course, you volunteer for an experiment that is attempting to do just that.

The Japanese neuroscientist Tomoyasu Horikawa and his colleagues used 'functional magnetic resonance imaging', or fMRI, which takes far more detailed images of brain activity than EEG does. By placing subjects in the scanner and waking them up around 50 times to ask them to report their dreams, the scientists built a bank of brain images correlated with dream reports. Eventually, researchers could read some of the content of their subjects' dreams merely by looking at the neural scans. Fortunately, in order to do this, the whole experiment must be repeated on each subject, given that brain activity is highly individual. In other words, scientists could not scan *my* brain 50 times and then read *your* dreams – so you don't have to worry about a research team sneaking into your bedroom and recording your dreams any time soon.

WHY DREAM?

WHAT DOES 'WHY' MEAN?

The question 'why do we dream?' is not as straightforward as it seems. That is because the answer to 'why' something happens can take several forms. I could mean 'why did I dream *last night*?'. That would require explaining why I fell asleep at a certain time and how my brain activated in a certain way. It might also involve explaining how my experiences during the day influence the types of dreams I have. This calls for a very complicated explanation. I might, instead, ask why I had a specific dream, or why I remembered that specific dream. Also complicated. A different 'why' question that has confounded scientists for decades is why humans dream at all. Is there an evolutionary explanation for dreaming?

ADAPTING TO PASS ON OUR GENES

We have good evolutionary explanations for many human features and their related abilities or 'traits', such as our ability to see with our eyes and hear with our ears. Evolution is all about *natural selection*. Living things, over many generations, have randomly occurring mutations that do not always affect their ability to survive. Often, however, mutations are disadvantageous or detrimental to survival and reproduction, making it less likely that the trait will be passed on.

Very occasionally, a mutation will be beneficial for survival and reproduction, meaning that trait is more likely to be passed on. A mutation that causes slightly better eyesight, for example, might be beneficial. The evolutionary story is much more complicated, of course, and there are many random factors. A small population with an extremely beneficial trait might happen to be living near a volcano that erupts, wiping out the population and the trait before it can be passed on. Alternatively, disadvantageous traits can be passed on if they are linked with a trait that is advantageous enough to outweigh the negative trait.

An example of this is back pain. Hominids developed the ability to walk upright some four to seven million years ago, which gave us significant advantages when living in a grassland environment. Our hands were freed up to use tools, and we could see over the tall savannah grass farther than quadrupeds could. However, an upright posture also puts great pressure on our lower backs. This is such a problem that back pain is the top contributor to disability worldwide. Meanwhile, this serious disadvantage is outweighed by the benefits of being bipedal, so the trait has not been adapted out of the population. Similarly, a trait that is neither advantageous nor disadvantageous may just stick around because it has never been adapted out, or because it comes with an advantageous trait. Given this complexity, are dreams adaptations or not?

We know more about the purpose of sleep than we

do about dreams. A variety of functions are carried out in the brain and body while we are resting, but there are still many mysteries, such as the specific functions of the different stages of sleep. There is no agreement at all, however, on the evolutionary function of dreams or on whether dreams even have a function.

DO DREAMS IMPROVE MEMORY?

When our bodies are resting and getting all the benefits of sleep, why do we have vivid hallucinations that intensely reactivate various areas of the brain? Sleep should be a well-deserved rest, not an exciting mental adventure, right? Some researchers think that this activation aids memory, which is very odd considering how bad our memories are, both 'in-dream' and 'post-dream'. How could dreams help memory? Two main functions that have been proposed are, firstly, that dreams *consolidate* memories and, secondly, that they *clear out* unnecessary memories.

For one thing, dreams may help us ensure that memories are stored well for the long term by actually replaying memories from the day while we sleep and strengthening their neural connections. This does not seem highly likely, though, because dreams do not just replay our waking experiences, and many bear no resemblance at all to our waking experiences. But perhaps dreaming happens *as a consequence* of the brain going through the process of strengthening these connections. Strong unconscious neural activation is required for memories to be put into long-term storage, and this also leads to conscious activation. Because the activation is somewhat random, our conscious mind then tries to make sense of it, generating dream narratives. In this view, the dream itself is not really an adaptive function but rather a consequence of the neural activation that provides the adaptive benefit.

Another option is that dreams might help us get rid of unnecessary memories. There could be a process that works in the same way as memory consolidation but in reverse. Research by a group of Japanese neuroscientists led by Akihiro Yamanaka suggests that REM sleep may serve this function in mice. If dreams replay memories as they get cleared out, this could also explain why they are bizarre. Removing memories is crucial, and those who remembered every bit of inconsequential daily information have a 'highly superior autobiographical memory', or HSAM – a rare and troubling condition diagnosed in about 60 people worldwide. It may sound quite nice to remember what happened on every single day of your life, but HSAM comes at a great cost.

In 2006, an American woman named Jill Price was the first person diagnosed with HSAM when she was in her early 40s. She finds the condition to be a heavy burden. Whenever a date is mentioned in conversation, on the television or on radio, all the details of that day come flooding back and her mind uncontrollably recites them until she is exhausted. Joey DeGrandis, who was diagnosed with the condition in his teens, a few years after Price, battles with depression and anxiety. Because he cannot forget, it is hard for him to move on after a bad experience: it is like everything *just happened*. In an interview, DeGrandis once explained that the memory of a breakup three years before was just as vivid in his mind, and the pain just as fresh, as if it had happened the day before – even though the relationship only lasted a few months.

It seems unlikely that consciously replaying events from the day would help us forget memories, but perhaps, as with the consolidation theory, dreams are simply a side effect of this process happening during REM sleep. Perhaps dreams occur both when we consolidate memories and when we delete them. This does not give dreams a function in themselves. Rather, they are a *consequence* of an adaptation. Even so, this would explain *why* we dream, although it is extremely difficult to confirm. Sleep itself plays an essential role in memory processing, but it remains unknown whether dreams are in any way related to this, either by processing the memories themselves or as a mere consequence of memory processing taking place.

FROM FREUD TO DARTS

Dreams may serve a different function other than helping with our cognitive processing. According to the *continuity hypothesis*, although we do not necessarily replay our waking experiences, dreams are in some way a continuation of waking life. They may play events out in a different way, mix experiences together or give us a chance to try out an alternative. This could serve several important functions. The famous Austrian neurologist and founder of psychoanalysis Sigmund Freud hypothesised that we dream about our true desires. During the day these are repressed by our conscious minds or 'superegos' because such thoughts are socially inappropriate and shameful. I won't go into too many details – which are inappropriate, after all – but you can look up the 'Oedipal complex' if you need an example. When we dream, some of these desires escape daytime repression.

However, dreams are usually indirect representations of our desires. The most terrible desires are dreamt of in symbols. Imagine – perish the thought – that I wanted to kill my best friend. This wish might be symbolised in a dream in which I chop off the heads of the roses in her garden. Other dreams might not be symbolic. Dreaming of eating lots and lots of cake is not necessarily a symbol, since the desire for yummy food is less shameful. Dreams can, therefore, serve two functions. One is just allowing us to let off steam by experiencing our desires come true in a safe, private environment where society will not judge us. Another is that we can analyse our dreams to work out what is bothering us, which can help us discover what we really want but are too repressed to admit. This requires a trained analyst, however, who can work out what the symbols mean. According to Freudian dream analysis, the symbols are specific to individuals and could not be as simple as, say, 'a dream about your teeth falling out means you have anxiety'. This dream would mean different things to different people and without an analyst, the meaning would remain obscure.

One reason to reject this symbolic view of dreams is

that we can have really disgusting, inappropriate dreams anyway, and they are quite common. Why would we symbolise some inappropriate desires and not others? Another problem with Freudian dream analysis is that some dreams seem so random they could mean just about anything, and there is no way to prove that one particular interpretation is correct.

If dreams are not continuous with waking, they could still be beneficial. According to the *discontinuity hypothesis*, the dreaming mind creates scenarios that are unlike waking, and this can serve a different set of functions. Dreams may give us scenarios where we can test out ideas or activities that have not occurred in real life. This could help us improve our creativity, and it seems that dreams do indeed serve this function for many artists and researchers. We can also practise movements in our dreams.

The German cognitive scientist Melanie Schädlich and her research group discovered that many professional athletes practise their sport while dreaming, which led her to wonder whether such practice is beneficial. She and her group devised an ingenious experiment to teach lucid dreamers to practise playing darts in their dreams. They found that those who managed to successfully practise several times showed more improvement in waking performance than those who did not manage to dream-practise. One view that this research supports is the *threat simulation hypothesis*, according to which our dreams create threatening scenarios that allow us to practise what we would do if they were to happen in real life. Imagine two ancient human ancestors: one who would regularly dream about escaping a woolly mammoth and one who could not dream. One day during a hunt, a mammoth attacks the group, and because the dreamer has had extra dream-practice, he survives and the other does not. This would mean our dreaming ancestor had an advantage, so dreamers would go on to have more children and pass on the dreaming trait. Schädlich's research suggests that dreams can improve performance, but threatening dreams may also help us make decisions faster or better when we are awake.

SPANDRELS OF THE MIND?

It is not clear, even if dreams *can* improve performance, whether this is actually their evolutionary function. An evolutionary adaptation must, at some point, have allowed a genetic mutation to be passed on more successfully than genes that do not carry the mutation. Most of the dreams I remember don't involve practising skills or scenarios, and it is unclear whether such dreams made my ancestors more capable of passing on their genes.

What if dreams serve no evolutionary purpose at all? Is that possible? Not all traits are adapted or selected for. According to *spandrel theory*, some human traits have not evolved due to natural selection but have piggy-backed on other traits that *are* useful. A 'spandrel' is that little triangular space on either side above an archway. The triangles themselves have no purpose. They are just a product of making the important parts. The keystone prevents the structure from collapsing and the pillars hold it up, but the spandrels are just there and if you take the stones out of them the arch will remain structurally intact. But artists often use spandrel spaces for paintings or carved reliefs that make it look nice.

Similarly, dreams may just be a consequence of having a conscious mind that spends quite a bit of its time sleeping, especially during REM sleep when a variety of brain functions are occurring. If dreams are the consequence of memory processing rather than part of the process, they would be mental spandrels. They could also be a consequence of some other cognitive process that occurs during sleep, or even just a random activation that is not a consequence of anything particularly useful. Dreams may just be 'cognitive trash' that occurs while the mind is trying to rest but is not entirely successful at doing so. Alternatively, what if dreams were actually a disadvantageous trait?

If dreams are disadvantageous, then they must have piggy-backed on something that is very important, like consciousness or memory consolidation. Such useful adaptations could counteract minor disadvantages caused by dreaming, allowing them to persist.

SLEEP DISRUPTION AND EMOTIONAL SPILLOVER

Dreams can disrupt sleep, which is bad for our health. Nightmares and thrilling dreams wake us up, and people who have repetitive nightmares can suffer severely. Lack of sleep is highly detrimental to our waking cognitive functions, so perhaps if we could have REM sleep with all of its assets but without dreams, that would be more beneficial. And besides disturbing our sleep, dreams can be downright upsetting.

Have you ever had a dream where someone was mean to you or your partner cheated on you and you stayed mad at them after you woke up? You may have known it was irrational but you were unable to shake off that betrayed feeling. This is very common and emotions can, apparently, spill over into waking life and affect relationships negatively. On the other hand, the opposite can also be true. Some people report having 'visitation' dreams in which deceased loved ones appear. Such a dream can give them the opportunity to say goodbye, ask forgiveness or forgive. Despite knowing that the dream was not real, people often feel they achieve closure from such dreams which may have a beneficial psychological effect.

As far as any evolutionary purpose goes, dreams are probably spandrels. I fail to see how, in our evolutionary past, dreams could have provided a significant benefit that would have actually allowed our ancestors to out-compete their non-dreaming cousins. Nevertheless, I do think dreams provide several non-evolutionary benefits: for one thing, they are really fun and incredibly interesting. But my main reason for finding dreams important is that they tell us an awful lot about human cognition, greatly benefiting the people who research consciousness and the mind.

HOW LITTLE WE AGREE

DO I KNOW MY OWN EXPERIENCES?

Despite all of the interesting findings in recent years, there are still many unsolved puzzles about dreams, but at least there is one thing we definitely know: people know what their own dreams are like. I wake up in the morning having just dreamt, and if I manage to keep hold of the memory, I would usually say I was just having a vivid hallucination and really thought I was awake at the time. Every once in a while, I'm lucky enough during the dream to realise that I'm dreaming and become lucid. These dreams are *exceptionally* vivid hallucinations. But am I so sure? If researchers can't even determine whether dreams are bizarre or not, then do we really know what they are like at all? Surprisingly, this particular issue is widely debated.

The most common view amongst researchers, and perhaps a plausible view for those of us who remember our dreams, is that dreams are hallucinations. So what does this mean? A hallucination is a type of perception that the mind creates, separate from reality. This can occur when the mind is shut off from the external environment as it is when we sleep. If dreams are hallucinations, then dreaming of looking at a tree would be the same type of experience as being awake and looking at a tree. Alternatively, a hallucination can occur when you are awake, for instance if hallucinogenic drugs make you see a dragon sleeping in a tree. The tree is real, but the dragon must be a hallucination.

There is good reason to believe that dreams are hallucinations because they seem so convincing and realistic. One could even say a dream can be 'hallucinated virtual reality', where we experience nearly all types of sensation, including movement. This is what led two German philosophers, Thomas Metzinger and Jennifer Windt, to present the idea in 2010 that dreams are "immersive, spatiotemporal hallucinations". What they mean, put simply, is that when we dream, we feel like we are *in* the dream, 'immersed' in the same way we feel immersed in reality while we are awake; that dreams involve the experience of movement in space and the passage of time; and that dreams are hallucinations which are *perceptual*.

What else could explain how realistic it feels to be in a dream? Sometimes things feel so real that it can take us a few minutes after waking to realise that it was all just a dream. When I dream about falling off my bike and wake up with my hands thrown out in front of me, it genuinely feels like I am falling, and it's always a huge relief to realise that it was just a dream. But others disagree, as Windt did in 2015, by then having done more research on how much sensations from the physical body affect what we experience in dreams. It turns out that dreamers feel far more real sensations than one might expect. Based on this, Windt proposed a slightly different theory about dreams from the one she and Metzinger had presented earlier. She now makes quite a convincing case arguing that dreams are actually illusions.

IT'S ALL AN ILLUSION

An illusion occurs when a real sensory experience is altered in some way so that our perception, although partly based on reality, is not accurate. Unlike a hallucination – which is perception in the absence of real sensation – an illusion is a modification of a real experience.

My favourite example is 'the pinwheel illusion'. You can try it out for yourself, as a quick Internet search will give you access to many online versions. The gist is that after looking at the centre of a rotating 'pinwheel' for one minute, you look away at something else, such as your hand, which will look like it is pulsating or even boiling. Windt thinks that since real stimuli are regularly felt while we are dreaming, many of the bodily sensations we experience in dreams are actually illusions of real bodily sensations. She regards these as illusions because they are real sensations that are misinterpreted as sensations coming from within the dream. One interesting misinterpretation of a bodily sensation, according to this view, occurs when we fall asleep. As our minds become less in touch with our bodies, it feels like we are actually falling. Therefore, my dream of falling off a bicycle could be explained not as a hallucination, but rather as an illusion of falling that is caused by me misinterpreting the feeling of 'falling' asleep.

This is quite similar to Aristotle's view that dream experiences are based on sensations, sounds, smells and perhaps even tastes that come from the dreamer's physical body. They 'filter into' the dream and are reinterpreted as sensations that are coming from *within* the dream. It is very unlikely, however, that everything we experience in our dreams is based on sensations that come from the external world. Sometimes light filters in, as I discussed earlier, but this does not give a good explanation of why we see the images we see when we dream.

Windt clarifies that unlike waking vision, which is based on bodily stimulus, dream vision is better described as hallucination, since it is very detailed. While we dream, our real eyes are closed, our physical surroundings are usually dark, and we will likely register light from the real world only occasionally, yet we still see vivid images. Since holding a picture or TV screen in front of a sleeping person's face is highly unlikely to cause them to dream about that image or TV footage, Windt reasons that our brains must generate the visual experiences in dreams without much help from real-world stimulus.

One problem with Windt's view – that most dream sensations are real sensations – is that it seems unlikely that sensation from the body would regularly match up with what we are doing in a dream. For example, if you reach out and grasp something, there might be a sensation of pressure on the grasping hand, but since your real hand is not grasping anything, there would be no real stimulus from your body. Experiments suggest that when sound stimulus infiltrates a dream, which only happens occasionally, our minds are quite good at incorporating it into the ongoing narrative or story, although this is often done in a weird way. Your alarm going off might sound like a baaing sheep, for instance, but it would be a strange-sounding sheep. And it would also be bizarre for a sheep to start baaing if you were dreaming of being in your office.

Fortunately, often the dreaming mind does not pick up on how outlandish these experiences are, and that may partially explain why dreams can be so incredibly odd. Yet since dreams are only sometimes weird in this way, it is not likely that regular infiltration by external stimuli can explain most dreams. If dreams are a mix of both hallucination and illusion, then they are still *perceptions* or experiences that feel like reality. But what if we are wrong about this too?

LET YOUR IMAGINATION SOAR

Perhaps dreams are more like *imagination*. And how, exactly, is this different from hallucination? Well, when we close our eyes and think about walking down the street in as much detail as possible, we can form a mental picture of doing so. It is often rather vague, although some people can form a fairly good mental image. Nevertheless, even clear, detailed imagination is not the same as hallucination. What do you think it would be like to close your eyes and suddenly start hallucinating that you were walking down the street? It would be shocking, and frightening too! Imagining, unlike hallucinating and sensory experience, is not perceptual. To me, dreams don't seem to be much like this at all. So why might a researcher think they are? Jonathan Ichikawa, who I mentioned earlier, argues that we do not really *believe* we are awake when we are dreaming. Perhaps we are just engrossed in the dream narrative and not paying attention to whether it is real or not. Or maybe we are only *dreaming* about believing we are awake. Even I, a fellow philosopher, find this reasoning a bit hard to wrap my head around.

A more scientific argument is that our ability to dream develops alongside our ability to clearly imagine and picture things in our head. This is the reason why Foulkes thought that we only develop the ability to dream after a few years, and that dreaming is not something that fetuses or even babies do. If the same cognitive mechanisms are required for both imagining and dreaming, but not for perceiving, this gives us good reason to think that dreaming is a type of imagining, not perceiving.

Daydreaming can seamlessly shift into dreaming, Ichikawa says. Think back to the last time you were letting your imagination wander and you fell asleep. Have you ever had a dream that followed along from this mind-wandering? Ichikawa argues that this is reason to think that dreams are just a more intense form of mind-wandering, as we do not really notice the difference when we shift between imagining and dreaming. Personally, I can't remember this ever happening to me, and I'm not convinced by this argument, given that our most vivid and realistic dreams occur during REM sleep and people don't usually go straight from a waking state into REM.

None of the theorists mentioned above are completely right or completely wrong, in my view. Rather, dreams involve all of these elements: sometimes they are more like hallucinations or imagination or illusion, and sometimes they are a mix.

Why are dreams so varied? The sleep stage we are in will strongly influence what kind of dream we have. It is likely that the dreams we have in NREM sleep are more imagination-like, and we are more likely to forget these dreams since they are less vivid, interesting and memorable. But during REM sleep, dreams are more hallucination-like and more vivid. It is even possible to mind-wander or imagine while having these dreams. However, sometimes we are more 'open' to illusions and sometimes more 'closed', depending on what stage of sleep we are in.

Dreams are very difficult to define and classify as one particular type of experience or another, which might partly explain why there is so much disagreement about what dreams essentially are. At this stage, however, my view is just a hypothesis, and we need to do a lot more research on dreams before we can pin them down.

TO SLEEP, PERCHANCE TO DREAM

DO ANYTHING, BE ANYONE

When I spring out of bed, terrified that I am about to get mauled by a lion that thirsts for my blood, it takes me a few moments to realise I am not in danger. I am in my bedroom, safe and sound. The fog slowly lifts from my mind and I realise how silly it was that I just thought I was about to die. That situation was so implausible – why didn't I realise it was a dream?

There are many fascinating mysteries about dreams that interest researchers and everyday people alike. Perhaps you get bored stiff listening to your friends tell you about their dreams, especially the long and elaborately detailed ones. Sure, they are really weird, but they don't follow any of the rules of a good story: they have no clear beginning, middle and end. They have no well-developed characters who must overcome some obstacle, just incongruous events that seemingly happen at random. And they have no consequences either. They are just poorly told, strange stories – yet you might want to listen to a dream report if the dream was about you.

Dreams are influenced by the waking world, just like Aristotle, that know-it-all, suggested all those thousands of years ago. Our dream selves feel real tactile stimuli, see real light and hear real sounds that come from the physical world. They can also affect our waking lives, and I might feel angry at you for being mean to me in my dream, even though I realise how irrational that is. You may believe that dreams are more meaningful than this if you are a follower of dream psychotherapy, such as Freudian analysis – and if your friends knew this, they probably wouldn't tell you about their dreams at all. Quite apart from that, some dreams are just too embarrassing to tell to anyone.

Many of us might find our dreams either too uninteresting or too personal to share with others, and yet, for ourselves, experiencing a dream is quite an amazing thing. It feels so real and is a phenomenon that no technology can currently replicate. The latest virtual reality or 'VR' systems involve putting on a headset and other gear that makes it look and feel like the wearer is somewhere else. A VR experience can be very convincing and realistic, and sometimes wearers even scream and shout in response to what they are seeing. If you would like to get a sense of how a VR headset works, you can download an app to your mobile and hold it up to your eyes to simulate this effect.

As a tech fix, VR is pretty cool, but it's not in the same league as dreaming. In a VR setup, as a wearer you always know that what you are seeing or experiencing is not real. In dreams, you really believe that you are there, touching, seeing, hearing and perhaps even tasting and smelling the environment. One day technology may catch up, rendering virtual landscapes so realistic that you forget they are unreal. But until then, the best way to experience genuinely convincing virtual reality is simply to fall asleep.

A RESEARCHER'S PLAYGROUND

Studying dreams is just as exciting as having them. Why do they have so many bizarre features? Why do they seem so real? Even the dullest dreams are actually fascinating. You are at your office, you make a phone call, nothing out of the ordinary happens. Yawn. But to a researcher, these might be the most interesting dreams of all. A mind largely shut off from the external world can simulate an office, the feeling of moving around, even having a conversation with a co-worker, with remarkable accuracy. Our decisions, behaviours and thoughts in such dreams can be quite normal. This is incredible, considering all of the chemical and activational changes the brain usually undergoes while we sleep.

We know about these chemical changes because of the great advances in sleep and dream research. Personally, I am impressed and thankful that so many scientists are willing to take up the challenge of studying dreams, even though it is extremely difficult. I am also grateful for the many study participants willing to serve as 'subjects' and have their brains scanned, their bodies tinkered with and their dreams – even the embarrassing ones – reported to a bunch of strangers in lab coats. Would you be willing to sacrifice your sleep and your privacy in the interest of furthering knowledge? Would you tell a scientist your most embarrassing dream? I love dream science, but I really love my sleep, too. On the other hand, wouldn't it be mind-blowing to be involved in a lucid-dream experiment and be taught how to control your dreams? Then you could do anything you want … if you successfully completed the experimental training.

Is it useful to dream? Perhaps. Having a dream about doing a task at the office may remind me of what I need to get done today, or alternatively it may suggest that I'm getting anxious at work. Maybe all the dreams I have about bikes will improve my cycling skills, just a little. Or maybe all of these dreams, the weird and the mundane ones, are improving my memory. Did dreaming help our ancient ancestors survive? This is very difficult to know, but if dreams do augment memory or improve skills, it could have been a benefit. Even if dreams were not an evolutionary advantage, they may be useful to individuals. I could dream of an idea for another book, or spend more time with my friends, although in dreams we would be able to fly around together. Have you always wanted to fly on a broom, like Harry Potter? Well, in your dreams you can. Harry could be there too, or you could even *be* Harry. Not even the sky is the limit, and if you want to, you can fly to the Moon.

When I think about my own dreams and how realistic they seem to be at the time, I feel sure that I know what it's like to dream. When I was afraid of being attacked by a lion, it was because I saw a lion, or at least I hallucinated that I saw a lion. But how sure am I that I wasn't just imagining a lion, like I do when I close my eyes and let my mind wander? Perhaps I'm not so sure after all. How do I know that the lion roaring wasn't just my alarm going off, or some sound coming from outside? This is very difficult to know unless I happen to wake up, hear the real sound and see where it's coming from.

What we know about dreams is fascinating, and what we have yet to discover about them is perplexing. One thing I do know is that studying dreams tells us a great deal about the human mind and about what it means to be conscious.